Introduction 2

   Diabetes: What is it? 4

   Hypos and Hypers: The difference between and how to treat both 5

   My Journey to Diagnosis 8

   Methods of Treatment Part 1: Carb Counting 10

   Methods of Treatment Part 2: Set Amounts 10

   Correction Doses (multiple dose insulin therapy) 12

   Food Substitutes 14

   5 reasons for eating 5 a day 19

   Closing Statement 23

   Table of References 23

Introduction

My name is Austin Jacobs and I have been a diabetic for a few months, so I am relatively new to it myself. I have been fortunate to be provided with a lot of knowledge and support in the preliminary stages of my journey through this life changing condition. Unfortunately, I know there are a lot of people out there without the type of support network that I have been blessed with, who will most likely be worried and confused at their new diagnosis. So, I thought to myself, I can help some of those people by passing on the knowledge I have obtained to make the preliminary stages of their journey a smooth transition to the world of diabetes.

It is important to note, that I am not, nor claim to be a medical professional, so before you take any of the advice on board make sure to consult a GP or diabetic specialist first, as I am just a 23-year-old type 1 diabetic so most of my advice can only come from personal experience. With that being said, I do hope that anyone who reads this can learn something about diabetes, whether it be for yourself as a newly diagnosed diabetic, you know someone who is diabetic or even just to expand your knowledge on an illness that everyone seems to know exists but know frighteningly little about.

This book will cover various topics, starting of course with an overview of what Diabetes actually is, and the different types of it. It is important to note however, that due to me being a type 1 diabetic, much of the book will be catered to those that are type 1. Some of the treatment methods and most, if not all, of the food substitutes that will be covered in this book will be applicable to type 2 diabetics as well.

We will go through what Hypoglycaemia and Hyperglycaemia are and how to treat both symptoms, backed up with proper guidance from the NHS website, because remember, I am not a doctor so a lot of the steps I have taken are available to find on the NHS website.

Diabetes: What is it?

Diabetes is a condition that causes a person's blood sugar level to become too high. (NHS Website, *Diabetes* 2023)

When being diagnosed with a lifelong condition, it can be daunting with the amount of information you get given. Above is a definition from the NHS website that describes in simple terms what diabetes is. Despite doctors' best efforts, there is no cure for diabetes, however if you are a type 2 diabetic, you can send it into remission where it has negligible effect on your daily life and overall health, providing it is kept in check.

There are 3 common types of diabetes; Type 1, Type 2, and gestational diabetes. Type 1 diabetes is where your body produces no insulin. This is because type 1 diabetes is an autoimmune condition, in where your body produces antibodies and sends them to attack the part of the pancreas that produces insulin, until there are no insulin producing cells left in the body. It is for this reason that type 1 diabetes can only be treated using insulin injections.

Type 2 diabetes is where your body does produce enough insulin, however you have a resistance to the insulin, making it not have the desired effect and in turn, raise your blood sugar levels. This form of diabetes is not an autoimmune condition and can be caused by several factors, including but not limited to;

- Living with obesity
- Too much abdominal fat stored around the liver or pancreas (in healthy people too)
- Genetic factors
- Living a sedentary lifestyle
- Diet
- Ethnicity

(Chapple, *What causes type 2 diabetes?* diabetes.com)

The best method of managing type 2 diabetes is through a healthy balanced diet and exercise. I have personally tried to aim to incorporate a large amount of protein to keep you full, usually about 1g per kg of bodyweight, but that can change depending on individual needs. I personally try to aim for between 8000-10000 steps of walking per day, however as that is not always possible, try to aim for at least 30 minutes of walking a day, ideally twice per day if time allows.

Gestational diabetes is the scientific term for being temporarily diabetic while pregnant, so this one is for the ladies. It is usually most common in the second or third trimester but can develop at any time during the pregnancy. It is usually most found in people over 40, who have 1 or both parents who are diabetic, and whose BMI is over 30. Those from ethnic backgrounds of Asian or African descent are also at increased risk. It is treated in the same way as type 2 diabetes, as one of the potential risks of gestational diabetes is if it not monitored correctly then can lead to permanent type 2 diabetes.

(NHS Website, *causes of gestational diabetes*)

Hypos and Hypers: The difference between and how to treat both

Hypoglycaemia and Hyperglycaemia are the two most drastic symptoms of diabetes to be on lookout for, as both can be fatal. Hypoglycaemia, or a Hypo for short, is where you blood sugar drops dangerously low, and requires immediate attention. The reason that a Hypo is so serious is because it can cause if you leave it untreated. Some of these effects include; Weakness and feeling sleepy, Seizures and fits, and collapsing or passing out. The main way of doing this is by giving your body fast-acting glucose, like sweets. In my experience I have found it good practise to always keep a bag of jelly babies on my person, as that way I always have a source of fast-acting glucose to have in the event of a Hypo. I usually take 3-5 jelly babies in the event of a Hypo, as any more than that can risk too much of a rise in the blood sugars and send you the other way. Like always though, it is best to ask your diabetic specialist or GP for the specifics, as they know your body better than I do. Another good method is to carry a small can of high sugar soft drink, preferably Lucozade. This is because it is easier for your body to process the glucose in a liquid than in solid food, as the body does not have to spend time digesting the liquid.

There are warning signs to a Hypo that you should look out for, and if you feel any of the warning signs then test your blood sugars immediately, as it can usually be treated by yourself if caught and prevent an unnecessary trip to the hospital. These signs include;

- sweating
- feeling tired
- **dizziness**
- feeling hungry
- tingling lips
- feeling shaky or trembling
- a fast or pounding heartbeat (**palpitations**)
- becoming easily irritated, tearful, anxious, or moody
- turning pale

(NHS Website, *Low Blood Sugar (Hypoglycaemia)*)

Once you understand what a Hypo is, a Hyper is the easiest thing to wrap your head around. Hyperglycaemia, or Hyper for short, is when your blood sugars spike higher than normal. This most commonly occurs after having carbs with a meal. While most people will not usually experience symptoms with a Hyper, it is important to recognise what the warning signs are so it can be treated, usually using an insulin injection. The biggest giveaway for me personally that my sugars are rising is I start sweating and feeling hot, however there are multiple others which include;

- passing more urine than normal, especially at night
- being very thirsty
- tiredness and lethargy
- thrush or other recurring bladder and skin infections
- headaches
- blurred vision
- weight loss
- feeling sick

If left untreated for a lengthened period, that is where the biggest concerns can arise with regards to a Hyper. The main health problem that such elevated bloods sugars can cause is damage to the nerves, particularly in your hands and feet. That is why you will usually have to have an annual appointment with a Podiatrist, or Foot Doctor. The effect of damaging these nerves is that you can lose the feeling in your hands and/or feet, making it difficult to grip thing or even to walk. (NHS Website, *High Blood Sugar (Hyperglycaemia)*)

So now you are caught up to speed about both Hypos and Hypers, it is time we take a little detour from the science stuff for a moment, and just delve into my journey from feeling generally fatigued, to how I became the latest diabetic in my family.

My Journey to Diagnosis

The journey to being diagnosed as a diabetic was one that was unexpected for me, but it was the best thing that could have happened as it answered a lot of questions. As a 22-year-old male, I always thought something was wrong about the levels of fatigue I was feeling, as well as the amount of water I was needing to drink to stay hydrated. I never thought to act on the suspicions that something could be wrong though, as I was working a manual labour job as a warehouse operative 8 hours a day, so I just put those symptoms down to that.

It was in work where the issue of potential diabetes was raised. You see I wanted to develop my skillset and increase my wages, in which that meant going in for my FLT licences. To achieve those, you first had to pass a medical examination. My eyesight, hearing and blood pressure came back fine; however, it was the urine sample that was the issue. The urine sample came back with exceedingly high concentration of glucose in it, so I was advised to contact my GP and arrange blood tests. This is where I was stupid, because I went into denial and thought I could just solve it by myself through diet and exercise, which would have helped had I been a Type 2 and not a Type 1.

A few months of work went by, and I went in for another medical, with the utmost confidence that I would pass it this time around. Safe to say, this was not the case, and once again the urine sample came back with a high concentration of glucose. On this occasion, I took a different approach and booked an appointment with my GP, who arranged for blood tests to be done. After a few days I was called into the doctors to discuss the blood tests, and for them to test my sugars in case it was a one-off occurrence. That test shown sugars so high up that they told me to go straight up to the hospital, where I spent 8 hours getting prodded with so many needles.

Ironically, I have always been afraid of needles in the past, which makes diabetes the worst possible illness to get really. You soon get used to it though, as I had the mentality of, I do not really have a choice otherwise I am going to end up ill. As of today, the needles and regular bloods being taken do not bother me anymore, and I am a better person in other areas of my life because of it. I am doing a lot more exercise, including weight training at least 4x per week, and playing football again. It has also made me realise the importance that diet has on your life, and that eventually, a bad diet will catch up with everyone.

Diabetes is a condition that will change a lot about you, how you think and how you choose to live your life and at first that can be extremely daunting to face, especially alone. It is important to note however that there are various people who you can go to for advice, such as your GP or diabetic consultant, and a lot of resources out there for you to read, like the NHS website or this book. The next few sections of the book will outline my 3 preferred treatments of Diabetes, and the best food alternatives as you look to switch to a more diabetic friendly diet, whilst still including the foods you love the most.

Methods of Treatment Part 1: Carb Counting

The first and most effective way for both types of diabetics to control their blood sugar levels is using carb counting. Carb counting does exactly what the name suggests, looking at the back of a packet or using an app like Nutracheck (my preferred choice of tracking app) to check how many grams of carbs are in the food that you are eating, and then applying a ratio to see how many units of insulin you need to take in order to keep your sugar levels in check. For most people, this ratio is usually a 1:10 ratio, so 1 unit of insulin for every 10g of carbs. Although this can differ, it can be a sign of insulin resistance if you deviate too much below that amount, which is more commonly a type 2 symptom. As an example, if you were to eat a Big Mac burger on its own, that contains 44g of carbs, so due to the second part being lower than five, you would round it down to 40g, which means you would need 4 units of fast acting insulin to counteract the carb intake and keep your blood sugar levels steady.

As carb counting is the most accurate method of controlling your blood sugar levels, most doctors and specialists prefer you to use this method. It is the most beneficial method that I have used, as it allows you a lot more flexibility in what you eat and when you eat. Do note however, that it does not allow for total freedom, and it is still important to eat everything in moderation as part of a healthy balanced diet. (NHS Website, *Eating a Balanced Diet* 2023)

Methods of Treatment Part 2: Set Amounts

Treating Diabetes using the set amounts method is easier to deal with when you first are diagnosed, as it means you are only taking insulin at certain times of the day, in certain doses advised by your diabetic consultant. It is used to provide a baseline for your consultant to analyse to see how the insulin affects your blood sugars when taken, so they can advise you accordingly on whether you will need more insulin than average. This method is extremely useful when you first are diagnosed, however in my opinion it is not sustainable long-term. The main factor in this is due to it restricting the times you can eat to the times you have your insulin, which for most people, is not an applicable method due to daily life, work commitments etc.

Particularly when you are first diagnosed with insulin, the set amounts will tend to be higher than what you will eventually take, as the main goal is to bring the blood sugars back in check as quickly as possible. However, it still must be done in a safe manner, so usually it is done to a certain ratio on how much insulin you can have per day as a maximum. The ratio for this is usually 0.55 x total body weight (in kg). So as an example, if your body weight were 100kg, you would do 100 x 0.55= 55 units of insulin per day. (University of California, *Calculating insulin dose* 2023)

This is why it is important to keep an eye on your weight as a diabetic and live a healthy lifestyle, as if you lose weight you need less insulin, so if you don't track your weight and keeping using the same amounts you can use too much and either end up in a hypo or end up overdosing.

Correction Doses (multiple dose insulin therapy)

Correction doses are an important thing when keeping you blood sugars at an optimum level. On multiple daily injections, there is more freedom as you do not need to plan so far in advance or be so restricted by injections delivered several hours ago. Because MDI involves rapid acting insulin, it has allowed people to wait less time before eating after injecting. Obviously, this depends on the overall glucose content of a meal, some people may be able to inject during or after a meal, without their blood sugar 'spiking' too much. Rapid acting insulin helps to reduce the effect of high blood sugar levels 1-2 hours after eating. (Singh, *Multiple dose injection (MDI) therapy, also known as multiple daily injections, is an alternative term for the basal/bolus regime of injecting insulin.* 2022)

Correction doses are best left though to once you are more confident in the level of insulin you need and managing your blood sugar levels. This is because there are some risks/disadvantages to using correction doses. These include but are not limited to;

- More chances of Hypos if administered incorrectly
- More risks being taken due to the increased freedom
- More chances of an overdose

Multiple daily injections should be accompanied by a strong understanding of how the regime works particularly as rapid acting insulin can lead to faster onset of hypos if dosing errors are made. A potential disadvantage of the extra freedom allowed by multiple daily injections can lead to more chances being take, such as eating types or quantities of foods that one would not eat on a twice daily regime. (Singh, *Multiple dose injection (MDI) therapy, also known as multiple daily injections, is an alternative term for the basal/bolus regime of injecting insulin.* 2022)

Food Substitutes

Looking after your diet is the number one most important thing when managing your blood sugar levels, as well as in the quality of life you can live on this earth. Sadly, not enough people realise this importance and as a result most people's knowledge on healthy diets is limited so they get stuck when diagnosed with something like diabetes that forces you to change your diet. Luckily, I have developed, through trial and error while training, 5 golden diet rules that I believe everybody, not just diabetics should follow.

1. Drink plenty of water
2. Prioritise Protein
3. Switch to complex carbohydrates
4. Have a portion of fruit/Vegetables with every meal
5. Track your Calories

people should aim to drink 6 to 8 cups or glasses of fluid a day. While there are many drinks, such as milk that is included in the 6-8 cups aim, I prefer to keep it to strictly water, as it is the best drink out there to keep your body hydrated, and trust me once your properly hydrated, you'll never go back. Also important for you to remember with this one, is that the 6-8 cup range is a base guideline, and you should 100% drink more than that if you're doing regular activity, whether that is in the gym, walking about places or working a manual labour job. There are many benefits to drinking enough water as well, which include;

1. It lubricates the joints

Cartilage, found in joints and the disks of the spine, contains around 80 percent water. Long-term dehydration can reduce the joints' shock-absorbing ability, leading to joint pain.

2. It forms saliva and mucus

Saliva helps us digest our food and keeps the mouth, nose, and eyes moist. This prevents friction and damage. Drinking water also keeps the mouth clean. Consumed instead of sweetened beverages, it can also reduce tooth decay.

3. It delivers oxygen throughout the body

Blood is more than 90 percent water, and blood carries oxygen to various parts of the body.

4. It boosts skin health and beauty

With dehydration, the skin can become more vulnerable to skin disorders and premature wrinkling.

5. It cushions the brain, spinal cord, and other sensitive tissues

Dehydration can affect brain structure and function. It is also involved in the production of hormones and neurotransmitters. Prolonged dehydration can lead to problems with thinking and reasoning.

6. It regulates body temperature

Water that is stored in the middle layers of the skin comes to the skin's surface as sweat when the body heats up. As it evaporates, it cools the body. In sport.

Some scientists have **suggested that** when there is too little water in the body, heat storage increases, and the individual is less able to tolerate heat strain.

Having a lot of water in the body may reduce physical strain if heat **stress** occurs during exercise. However, more research is needed into these effects.

7. The digestive system depends on it

The bowel needs water to work properly. Dehydration can lead to digestive problems, **constipation**, and an overly acidic stomach. This increases the risk of **heartburn** and stomach ulcers.

8. It flushes body waste

Water is needed in the processes of sweating and removal of urine and faeces.

9. It helps maintain blood pressure

A lack of water can cause blood to become thicker, increasing **blood pressure**.

10. The airways need it

When dehydrated, airways are restricted by the body to minimize water loss. This can make **asthma** and allergies worse.

11. It makes minerals and nutrients accessible

These **dissolve in water**, which makes it possible for them to reach various parts of the body.

12. It prevents kidney damage

The kidneys regulate fluid in the body. Insufficient water can lead to kidney stones and other problems.

(Medical news today, *15 benefits of drinking water and other water facts* 2023)

The second rule is to prioritise protein. The recommended daily amount of protein is 0.8g per kg of bodyweight. However, I say try to aim slightly higher than that as then if you fall short you're still getting enough protein in to stay healthy. A lack protein in your diet will lead to a range of health concerns. These can include skin lesions, thin brittle hair and hormone imbalances. On a long-term basis, low protein intake may lead to a condition known as sarcopenia. This is the loss of muscle mass during the ageing process. A lack of muscle mass in an older person can be quite debilitating as it can prevent day to day activity that can be taken for granted at a younger age. (Agnew, *How much protein do I need?: MYPROTEIN™* 2021)

You do have to be careful not to intake too much protein however, so balance is key. Too much protein can have adverse effects on the body, as stated in the below excerpt from Myprotein.com.

"Over the years, the safety of high protein intakes has been heavily discussed. Whilst a lot of negative reports of high protein intakes have been proven to be unfounded in healthy individuals, those with existing health conditions (especially kidney problems) should exercise caution and discuss with a doctor or a registered dietician before starting a high protein diet.

For healthy individuals there is evidence that long term intakes as high as 3.4.4g/kg/d have no detrimental health impacts. However, if you take your protein intake up too much and in any way that will prevent you from getting in enough other macronutrients whilst sticking to your calorie allowance may cause problems. For example, if you are having so much protein that you do not have enough calories left for an appropriate amount of carbohydrates, side effects may include constipation, dehydration, and bad breath.

Eating a balanced diet with a protein intake optimal for your health and fitness goals (1.2-2-5g/kg/d) will help to reduce side effects and prevent health concerns."

(Agnew, *how much protein do I need?: MYPROTEIN™ 2021*)

The third rule is to switch to more complex carbohydrates. This is useful for a diabetic as we want to try and limit how much our blood sugars spike after eating a meal, and complex carbohydrates do just that. Being loaded with more fibre than regular carbohydrates, the complex versions of the foods take longer for our body to digest, promoting better digestive health and meaning the body cannot access the glucose as quickly. This in turn stops the spike being as severe as the insulin you would have taken before the meal has time to get into your bloodstream and use up any existing glucose before more gets put into the body. Some examples of complex carbs that I recommend are as follows;

- Sweet potatoes
- Brown rice
- Brown pasta
- Brown bread
- Oats
- Pumpkin

- Kidney beans

The fourth rule is having a portion of fruit and veg with every meal. Fruit and vegetables are part of a healthy, balanced diet and can help you stay healthy. It's important that you eat enough of them.

Evidence shows there are significant health benefits to getting at least 5 portions of a variety of fruit and vegetables every day. That's 5 portions of fruit and veg in total, not 5 portions of each. A portion of fruit or vegetables is 80g.

The 5 A Day campaign is based on advice from the World Health Organization (WHO), which recommends eating a minimum of 400g of fruit and vegetables a day to lower the risk of serious health problems, such as heart disease, stroke and some types of cancer.

5 reasons for eating 5 a day

6. Fruit and vegetables are a good source of vitamins and minerals, including folate, vitamin C and potassium.
7. They're an excellent source of dietary fibre, which can help to maintain a healthy gut and prevent constipation and other digestion problems. A diet high in fibre can also reduce your risk of bowel cancer.
8. They can help to reduce your risk of heart disease, stroke and some types of cancer.
9. Fruit and vegetables contribute to a healthy, balanced diet.
10. Fruit and vegetables taste delicious and there's so much variety to choose from.

Fruit and vegetables are also usually low in fat and calories (provided you do not fry them or roast them in lots of oil). That's why eating them can help you maintain a healthy weight and keep your heart healthy. To get the most out of your 5 A Day, your 5 portions should include a variety of fruit and vegetables. This is because different fruits and vegetables contain different combinations of fibre, vitamins, minerals and other nutrients. Almost all fruit and vegetables count towards your 5 A Day. They can be fresh, frozen, canned, dried or juiced. Potatoes, yams and cassava do not count because they mainly contribute starch to the diet.

(NHS website, *why 5 a day?* 2023)

The fifth and last rule is to track your daily calorie intake. Being obese can lead to all sorts of problems with regards to diabetes, and the best way to avoid becoming obese is to track your daily calorie intake and make sure you do not go above your maintenance calories for most of the time. It takes an excess of 3500 calories on top of your daily amount to gain 1lb of fat, so it's hard to do unless you're continually eating.

The main question on your mind right now is how you calculate your daily calorie intake. While you can just use the reference amount for an adult, which is around 1600 for women and around 2000 for men, I do not recommend this. Instead, I recommend going online to a calorie calculator to calculate the exact amount or multiplying your weight in lbs by 15. This is to ensure maximum accuracy.

Tracking your calories is a vital aspect of preventing weight gain and maintaining a healthy lifestyle. By monitoring your caloric intake, you gain valuable insights into your eating habits and can make informed decisions about your diet. Here are a few reasons why calorie tracking is crucial in preventing weight gain:

- Awareness: Calorie tracking raises your awareness of the energy content in the foods you consume. It helps you understand portion sizes and the calorie-dense nature of certain foods. This knowledge enables you to make conscious choices and avoid mindless overeating.
- Accountability: Tracking your calories holds you accountable for what you eat. It helps you stay on track with your dietary goals and promotes a sense of responsibility. When you know you have to record your food intake, you are more likely to make healthier choices and resist temptation.
- Balancing Energy: Weight gain occurs when there is an imbalance between calorie intake and expenditure. By tracking your calories, you can strike a balance by adjusting your food choices and portion sizes to meet your energy needs. It allows you to create a calorie deficit if weight loss is your goal or maintain a calorie balance to prevent weight gain.
- Identifying Patterns: Calorie tracking helps identify patterns in your eating habits. You can observe whether certain foods or situations lead to overeating or excessive calorie consumption. Recognizing these patterns empowers you to make necessary changes and develop healthier eating behaviours.
- Motivation and Progress: Monitoring your calorie intake provides a tangible way to measure your progress. Seeing the numbers and observing positive changes can be highly motivating. It allows you to celebrate achievements, stay focused, and make necessary adjustments to reach your weight management goals.

In summary, tracking your calories plays a pivotal role in preventing weight gain by increasing awareness, promoting accountability, balancing energy, identifying patterns, and providing motivation for positive change. Embracing this practice empowers you to take control of your diet and make informed decisions that contribute to a healthier and happier you.

Closing Statement

I would like to take the time to thank you for reading this book to the very end, it has been a pleasure to share the knowledge passed onto me as a newly diagnosed diabetic and hopefully, the knowledge you have learned throughout this short book will help you in your diabetic journey. Just always remember that there are people out there to talk to if you are struggling with your new diagnoses, and you never have to suffer alone.

References

15 benefits of drinking water and other water facts (2023) *Medical News Today*. Available at: https://www.medicalnewstoday.com/articles/290814#benefits (Accessed: 26 June 2023).

Agnew, L. (2021) *How much protein do I need?: MYPROTEINTM, MYPROTEIN*. Available at: https://www.myprotein.com/thezone/nutrition/how-much-protein-do-i-need/?thg_ppc_campaign=71700000079906104&product_id&gclsrc=3p.ds&affil=mpppc&gclid=04bce1161bd71657b465858c173e2b98&msclkid=04bce1161bd71657b465858c173e2b98&utm_source=bing&utm_medium=cpc&utm_campaign=UK+%7C%7C+EN+%7C%7C+SEA+%7C%7C+DSA+%7C%7C+NB+%7C%7C+The+Zone&utm_term=%2Fthezone%2Fnutrition%2F&utm_content=Core+-+Zone+%7C%7C+Nutrition (Accessed: 26 June 2023).

Calculating insulin dose (2023) *Diabetes Teaching Center*. Available at: https://diabetesteachingcenter.ucsf.edu/calculating-insulin-dose/ (Accessed: 26 June 2023).

Singh, A. (2022) *Multiple dose injection (MDI) therapy, also known as multiple daily injections, is an alternative term for the basal/bolus regime of injecting insulin., Diabetes*. Available at: https://www.diabetes.co.uk/insulin/multiple-dose-insulin-injection-therapy.html (Accessed: 26 June 2023).

Website, N. (2023a) *Eating a Balanced Diet, NHS choices*. Available at: https://www.nhs.uk/live-well/eat-well/how-to-eat-a-balanced-diet/eating-a-balanced-diet/ (Accessed: 23 June 2023).

Website, N. (2023b) *What is Diabetes, NHS choices*. Available at: https://www.nhs.uk/conditions/diabetes/ (Accessed: 26 June 2023).

why 5 a day? (2023) *NHS choices*. Available at: https://www.nhs.uk/live-well/eat-well/5-a-day/why-5-a-day/ (Accessed: 26 June 2023).

www.ingramcontent.com/pod-product-compliance
Lightning Source LLC
Chambersburg PA
CBHW082125220526
45472CB00009B/2306